A short

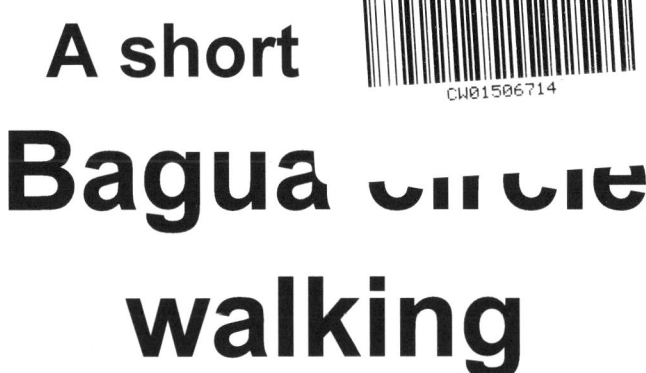

Bagua circle walking

by Edward Hines

ISBN 1519250312

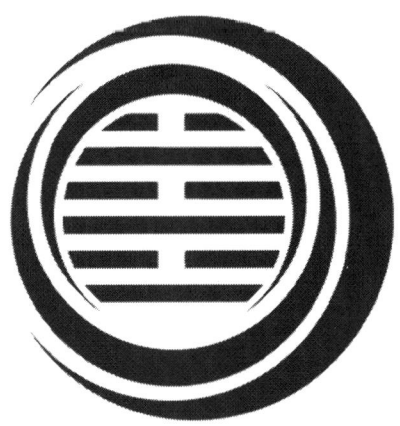

Disclaimer

I have included the following paragraphs as a sad necessity of our times, to which I reluctantly bow. Responsibility for your own actions should be a given.

The techniques, ideas, and suggestions in this book are not intended as a substitute for proper medical advice. Martial arts and other forms of exercise can be dangerous, especially if performed without proper pre-exercise evaluation, competent instruction and personal supervision from a qualified fitness professional.

Always consult your physician or health care professional before performing any new exercise, exercise technique or beginning any new diet—particularly if you are pregnant, nursing, elderly, or if you have any chronic or recurring conditions.

Any application of the techniques, ideas, and suggestions in this document is at the reader's sole discretion and risk.

The editors, authors and publishers of this book are not liable or responsible to any person or entity for any errors contained in this book, or for any special, incidental, or consequential damage caused or alleged to be caused directly or indirectly by the information contained within.

Dedication

To Alan, who knew the meaning of dedication.

Other books by Edward Hines

Beginning Bagua

Moving into Stillness

Coming soon:

Single palm change – a guide to Baguazhang's key movement

The book of Baguazhang basics – big, beautiful and bulshit – free

The applied circles of Baguazhang

Table of Contents

Introduction

Circle walking has been a part of my life since I first met Luo Dexiu in Taiwan over 24 years ago. Circle walking has been a riddle, a comfort, a source of strength, of calm, a burden, a joy and many other things. I cannot say that I have never missed a day in that time. I've missed quite a lot of days. But I've always come back, and there has always been more waiting for me.

When I started *Baguazhang* there was little written or video material available on the subject. Much of it was misleading one way or another, too mystical, too vague, too promotional. These days there is a lot more information readily available.

However more is not always good. Yes I'm fully aware of the irony of me adding to that more. I want to write a short and practical book a little in the spirit of a *sanda* classmate of mine who said of the *Taiji* classics 'People read all kinds of mystical stuff into the *Taiji* classics, I prefer to think of them more as a manual, like a manual for driving a car.'

In this book I use the words *Bagua* and *Baguazhang* interchangeably. I realise that without context this is not entirely correct, however it matches my spoken usage and has not caused confusion as far as I know.

About circle walking

Circle walking is the core practice of *Baguazhang*. It is not the only practice, and you cannot get everything from it as some teachers might suggest. However since it is really key to so many aspects of *Baguazhang* it's a good idea to be clear about how to practise.

What makes *Baguazhang* special, in relation to many preceding Asian martial arts is that it is based on natural human locomotion. Most Asian martial arts put a lot of emphasis on fixed stances, *bu*, though experienced martial artists understand that it is the transition into the stance that gives the stance function (and the Chinese character for step and stance are the same).

In *Baguazhang* the emphasis is much more in the transitions than the fixed shapes.

Everyone knows how to walk, right? Well more or less, and *Baguazhang* goes deeply into the conscious exploration of walking to develop valued qualities.

What circle walking can do for you:

- Provide a centering, calming, refreshing moving meditation

- Improve body awareness, posture, balance and agility
- Strengthen your legs, aspects of mobility and improve your balance
- Develop your martial power
- Explore strategic and tactical movement
- Create a sense of 'ownership' of the space around the body

What makes circle walking so appealing once you have developed it as a skill is the feeling of flow, the ability to remain increasingly stable in motion, to be both solid and sensitive, of being simultaneously unstoppable and able to change fluidly.

Another important aspect of circle walking as exercise is that it combines what are often contradictory elements — calmness and activity. For the body to maximise its natural healing abilities it needs to be calm. Another important component of healing you is circulation of blood and lymph, and these circulations are stimulated by the act of walking.

Of course this takes practise, and it can be a demanding practise. Circle walking requires mobility through the joints of the legs, strength, balance and control. Fortunately it also develops these qualities.

While it may be useful for many people to do some prior work before beginning to circle walk, the approach I want offer here is starting easy, and gradually adding in difficulty.

What circle walking includes

- Weight transfer, weight transfer, weight transfer
- Circle walking is moving in a straight line (ok a curved one)
- Circle walking is changing directions
- Circle walking is kicking, trapping and throwing

A useful I rule to remember when you practise is that *you can't do it all at once,* at least to start.

Practice is the gradual layering in of different qualities and abilities. To start with pick a single quality or ability and focus on it, until it becomes largely automatic.

Practice can be more than just the development of physical skills and qualities. You might ask how can it not be more?

When you start to circle walk, you are training mental or emotional qualities in a very real way. You are also tracing a shape that is held in reverence by many traditions the world over, a shape that has metaphoric as well as geometric qualities.

How and whether you choose to engage with these other meanings of circle walking is a personal choice. The emphasis in this book is as concretely on the physical, though that does not mean that is all there is.

Pay more attention to quality than volume of practice. The quality of your practice is determined by your ability to focus on what matters.

Knowing what matters is a different challenge. It is usually the role of the teacher to help you find the most useful focus, and there is no real replacement to a live teacher. Still I will do my best in this book to help you determine what you need to focus on.

The structure of this book

This book has a number of distinct sections. Many of these refer to Gao Yisheng's writings on *Baguazhang*.

The first describes the general body requirements of circle walking, from head to toe, from inside to outside.

The next section illustrates the most important hand and body positions that you can use for circle walking.

The third section outlines different ways to structure your practice. It includes a logical order of development, images and partner exercises.

Read over the book, use it as a reference, and most importantly apply it to your practise.

This book does not go into palm changes or the use of *Baguazhang* as a martial art. I refer you to my other books, and my website if you want further instruction on these aspects of *Baguazhang*.

The challenge of Chinese martial arts books

Chinese martial arts books have certain common characteristics, that relate to their culture and subculture of origin. Chinese culture reveres the old, Chinese martial arts culture tends to hide what is important, and finally Chinese martial artists do not like to lose face.

Concretely this means that when a writing, a rule or idea is embedded in the culture it is rarely questioned. In Chinese martial arts certain verses of explanation have become embedded. The original meaning can be lost, but the parroted phrase is explained to fit the understanding of generations that have not quite 'got it.'

The speed of distortion is doubled when you throw in western and new age attempts to fit what are essentially tips on body control into a swirled qis (rather than whirled peas) cosmic perspective.

Most often the phrases can be understood in simple terms. Often there are redundancies. Redundancies have three main sources. The first is this 'I'm going to repeat this because it's important and you probably won't get it first time, or the second, or the third...'

The second is 'Hey, that school uses these classic verses, we better had too or we'll be seen as ignorant.'

The third is that teachers sometimes charge by the line. I mean that literally, many teachers in the past charged per line of song, with accompanying technique/explanation. Not so different from charging by the form. This also goes *some* way to explaining the proliferation of forms in many Chinese martial arts schools.

By using Gao Yisheng's writings as a guide for this book I have gone some way towards falling into the 'the others all talk about this I better had too' trap. I hope that I do it in a down to earth enough way that you will not waste too much time getting lost in esoterica.

Here is a standard for you to consider next time you read a *Bagua* book and feel confused or insecure due to lack of understanding. Ask yourself if the writer trying to explain, or to create and maintain a sense of superiority?

Of course there are things that you do not understand *yet*, however this is a physical art and explanations *can be graspable.* Each graspable instruction can provide a firmness that allows you to explore and map the emptiness around it.

I have a great deal to thank my teacher Luo Dexiu for. He sets a fine example for lucid and demonstrable explanations.

What you will not find in this book

Some people will buy this book looking for certain pieces of information that they will not find. I'll divide these 'missing pieces' into two categories.

The first is very detailed bio-mechanical descriptions of the postures and movements, or a detailed 'energetic' description.

The second category is martial applications and techniques.

Leaving these out is a deliberate choice. For readers who tend towards a feeling of disappointment here I suggest you take Rumi's advice 'the sign of a sufi is joy at sudden disappointment'.

You bought this book because you thought you could learn something from the author. This section might contain the most valuable ideas for you.

I do not provide details of bio-mechanics or 'energy' in part because it is very difficult to convey these in a book.

More importantly even if I did I have no idea of the state of your body or emotions. Any prescription I gave you could be the wrong one.

In the same vein the idea of practise is to know your own body. This is a personal process. It may need a little push to start, a process to use as the laboratory for investigation. However if I gave 'end results' in the form of some complex visualisation of energy or fiddly description of joint angles then many readers would distort their movements in the desire to conform to the instructions.

There is a third reason which I'll remain cryptic about. You can ask me in person.

So follow simple instructions of process, develop your living awareness and you'll get something more valuable than 'the *qi* goes here then it goes here;'

Now to explain the lack of martial applications.

There is a hunger among many *Bagua* practitioners to understand how to apply forms. I understand this because so many forms seem so abstract until you develop the eye to read them. I also appreciate the desire to be able to focus on a clear martial use to avoid the degeneration to empty choreography that is so common in *Taiji*.

However I will not present any applications because I want readers to consider a movement approach to *Baguazhang*.

When I first met Luo Dexiu one of the things that stood out the most was the quality of his movement. The movements themselves were interesting, and the class I observed was full of striking, controlling and throwing applications.

However what I appreciated most was Luo's movement, his ability to remain in balance in himself which allowed him to move with a frightening speed for a big man, then to arrive where he wanted with his entire body, and to change direction with a deceptive smoothness.

I leave out applications because I want to underline this aspect of practise. How do you use these instructions to improve your quality of movement, to integrate the limbs with the trunk? Can you use your *Baguazhang* to better understand movement, the relation between one part of your body and other parts of your body?

When you understand this, when you can move well, techniques become easy. But if you focus on techniques as an end in themselves your risk becoming brittle, predictable and limited in your movement.

Body use in circle walking

The guidelines below come from Gao Yisheng's writing. They are presented slightly out of order as I have divided them into sections relating to different parts of the body.

Obviously you can circle walk in different ways. The rules below are somewhat flexible, in that they must be adapted to different arm positions and stepping methods. The instructions refer most clearly to the well known circle walking posture below.

Figure 1. Turning palm – the well known circle walking posture

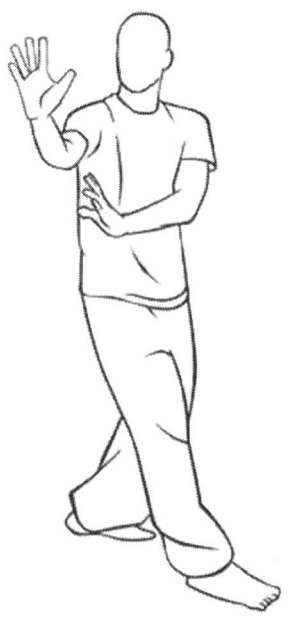

After the general descriptions in this section I will go on to describe various ways to structure practise, the intentions and effects behind them.

Remember that each individual line or instruction points not just to a section of the body, but to a part of the whole. The goal is to create a body that is connected but flexible, a relationship between the joints that allows the weight and movement of the body (power) to be focused at any point easily without excess stiffness or tension.

Sculpt your own Bagua body

Imagine I give you a big block of marble, a hammer and chisel and ask you to sculpt your body in the posture above. Where do you start? With your face? With your hair? With your fingers?

I don't think so. You probably would not add in details until you had carved out the approximate shape. Once you've done this, then you can gradually add in detail.

In a similar vein, when undoing the nuts on a wheel to change the tyre you loosen each nut a little at a time rather than unscrewing one completely and finding the other three have taken up the tension and become stuck.

It's not that the details are not important, but they do not become important until the crude shape is in place.

So read through all the instructions below, get the basic idea, then piece by piece add in more awareness, more attention and more detail a little at a time.

Breath

In our school the first two principles stated for circle walking are

1. 意要靜 The mind must be peaceful.

2. 氣要平 One's Qi should be smooth.

So I want to start with the breath. Not because by developing your *qi* you will gain invincibility and a few magic powers, simply because it is an efficient route to develop a calm mind and the body awareness needed to work on the other qualities.

The simplest way to think of these two lines is that circle walking should not be an emotional matter. It's not a question of forcing yourself into brow furrowed concentration at each step. A better idea to think of it as a stroll in the park.

If you are already calm enough, then great. If not you can play with a few options.

The first is to walk briskly without much attention to detail. I know it sounds very Victorian, but a vigorous stride can work wonders on the mood. It's not just me who believes this, plenty of studies show this to be the case.

If you already have a degree of emotional tranquility you may notice that a smooth breath and a calm mind go together. You can cultivate the two deliberately.

Here is a method that helps.

1. Observe your breath while in an upright posture of some kind, whether seated or standing.

2. On the inhalation, feel your lower abdomen, allow the belly to expand. Keep your mind and attention gentle – do not force the breath, encourage it.

3. Let the breath stay as long as it needs, when you exhale observe the sense of relaxation that comes with it.

4. Pay attention to your body while you wait for the next inhalation.

This method is super simple, if not always easy. If you practise this regularly it will become easier and easier to enter a calm and focused state.

The emphasis on the belly is useful as this also happens to be your centre of gravity. If you are relaxed and aware of your centre of gravity it is far easier to remain balanced in movement.

When you start to circle walk and do other kinds of *Bagua* exercises you want the movements to be supported by your centre of gravity. It helps to have easy access to awareness of this area.

Finally when you circle walk while breathing this way the sensations can be highly agreeable. I will not try to describe them here, much better you find out for yourself. You will know.

Still don't limit yourself to easy success, or build too much into agreeable sensations. They come, they go and there is always more. It's just a good place to start.

The head

The following guidelines for the head are fairly straightforward, and common across many Chinese martial arts.

3. 頭要頂 The head should be erect.

4. 舌要抵 The tongue should touch the roof of the mouth.

5. 項要挺 The neck should be held straight.

6. 眼要隨 The eyes should follow.

Let's start with the head being erect. The head is one end of your spine, and if it is out of line it will affect your entire posture, your ability to move freely and your ability to manage external forces.

To place your head is relatively simple, though there are some errors you can make. Essentially you can imagine the top of your ears being pulled gently upwards. The front of the neck should lengthen. The chin should tuck slightly as a result of the head lifting, rather than by deliberately pulling inwards.

Do not force your head up. Many people have heads that chronically slump forwards, due to sedentary lifestyle, computer and mobile phone use.

This is not something that you can change overnight. You will not be able to force your head into place. The more hours per day you can gently improve your head posture the better — within reason. The head was made to be moved as well, the basic position is upright, but you should also be able to look up down, left right and glide in any direction.

Obviously the position of the head depends on how you hold the neck, and if your head is in the correct position, your neck will be too. If you want to focus on your neck specifically, then maintain a balance between pushing the rear of the neck backwards, and, lengthening the front of the neck. Generally in circle walking the head may twist (rotate in medial plane) but does not tilt in the frontal or sagittal planes.

The tongue touching the roof of the mouth has several functions. The first is that it stops you biting your tongue - a real risk if you are struck with your tongue between your teeth.

The second relates to pressure and connection in the body. Lifting the tongue connects the front line of the body to the posterior line of the body. Take a deep belly breath with the tongue up, and the tongue down. You can feel the difference in how the tongue position changes the sense of pressure and stretch along the front of the body.

The third use is that the tongue can act as a kinesthetic pointer which directs awareness to key points in the brain used in *Daoist* meditation. That is a little beyond the scope of this book.

The next question is what do the eyes follow and how? Eye movement can be both indicative and causative of excessive mental activity. So to calm the mind it is helpful to keep the eyes relatively stable and fixed in position.

When circle walking in the well known *Bagua* guard position the eyes gaze towards the tip of the index finger of the raised hand (some schools will choose the space between the thumb and index finger, or some other minor variation). This serves to fix the gaze, and as the hand moves through a change the eyes follow.

There is not always a clear gaze point in many of the postures. In which case the eyes will be level and straight forward. Following in this case refers to being receptive, allowing vision to enter, rather than actively seeking out things to look at. This receptive vision is mentally calming and also tends to help create greater peripheral awareness. Peripheral vision is adept at detecting movement, which is useful for a martial art.

The torso

7. 田要抱 Hold the *dantian*.

8. 肛要提 Lift the anus.

9. 肩要垂 The shoulders should hang down.

10. 肘要墬 The elbows should sink.

11. 胸要含 The chest should be collapsed.

When you first read the list pertaining to the torso some instructions can seem strange and ambiguous. I have certainly seen some explained and interpreted bizarrely. In fact these instructions are relatively simple and all point towards a means of maintaining a unified body.

As I said earlier though you can focus on individual lines of these instructions, that is partly a result of the medium in which they are presented – words rather than movements. So each time you read through one section of these instructions use what you learn to enrich the mental image of the entire body.

Strictly speaking the elbows are not part of the torso, I included the instruction here because the elbows and shoulders are closely related, and the goal of the practice is to unify the body -[***] to see how each part connects to and is affected by the other parts.

So what do these lines point to? A state of the body in which it feels full and connected – a positioning of the shoulders relative to the spine which allows the torso to apply force into the arms with minimal shoulder tension.

The sections starts with two lines about the *dantien* and lower abdomen. The two lines go together, and refer to sitting down gently into the posture. The sitting down is what 'lifts' the anus and the resultant shape is what holds the *dantien* – in this case the entire lower abdomen rather than a single point.

Figure 2. Holding refers to the seated posture, not the position of the hands

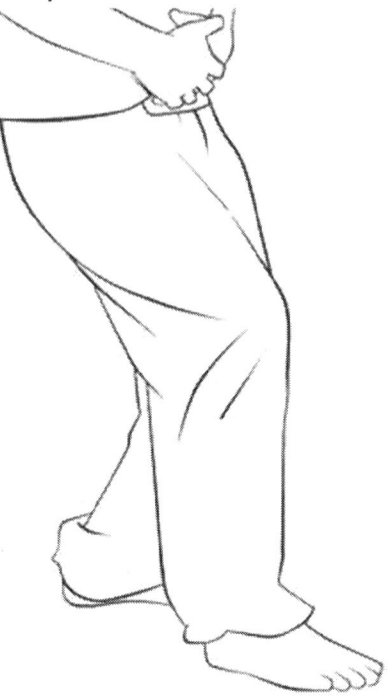

Holding the *dantien* means keeping some tension and attention in the lower abdomen, to not simply let the belly sag out on each inhalation. The tension should be light. This line also relates to the line below.

The advice about the anus is often misinterpreted. The anus and perineum form the lowest part of the *dantien*. A small degree of muscular tension here is a part of holding the dantien. Also this area engages naturally if you prepare to squat or jump.

There is no need to walk like a toddler desperately trying to keep one in, or to tuck the hips in a posterior tilt as is sometimes talked about. OK the first one is never suggested as far as I know, though many people do think they need to be more tense at the level of anus and perineum than necessary.

Holding the *dantien*, which includes its lower limits in the perineum and anus allows the practitioner to deliberately adjust the fluid pressure in the body via the breath (this is an aspect of qi).

Attention to the *dantien* in this way facilitates awareness of the centre of mass of the body, and it's role in maintaining balance as well as generating force. If you can move your centre of gravity lightly and efficiently, the rest of the body will be easier to control and place.

Now let's consider the top side of the torso.

The shoulders hanging down are a complement to the head pushing up. You allow your shoulders to relax down, by relaxing the upper trapezius muscles and allowing the shoulder blades to sink down the back. This creates a gentle stretched connection along the sides of the head and neck to the arms.

A relaxed shoulder moves more easily than a tense one, and it allows force from the body to be propagated into the arm without blockage.

Collapsing the chest really means not lifting it, or pushing it forward. In most *Bagua* postures the hands and elbows are held in ahead of the frontal plane, and thus ahead of the chest. This makes the chest 'collapsed' or hollow relative to the arms.

Equally importantly allowing the chest to stay relaxed downwards emphasizes the use of the back in transmitting force to the arms.

The back 'pushes' through the shoulders, down to the elbows and eventually to the hands.

To facilitate this the elbows point downwards where possible, and drop to the lowest position that they can relative to the hand and shoulder.

Rotating the point of the elbow upwards also tends to make the shoulder lift, which contradicts the idea of sinking the shoulders.

Sinking the elbow is a way to guide force from the body so that it is not lost in a elbow that buckles or twists.

A slightly bent elbow is less vulnerable to being broken, and elbows can be used to protect the body from blows combined with the fore and upper arms.

The hips

12. 腰要擰 Twist the waist.

13. 胯要坐 Sit into your hips.

The order of these two lines makes more sense reversed. The Chinese word hips refers to the inguinal fold of the hips. Sitting into the hips means bending the knees as if to sit on an imaginary stool, as such it relates to the first two lines referring to the torso.

By sitting into the hips it is much easier to twist rotate the waist horizontally because it is easier to differentiate the rotation of each hip and its role in turning the hips. Don't over think this one, just try it out and you'll see it's simple.

Figure 3 – 1. stand, 2. sit, 3.then twist

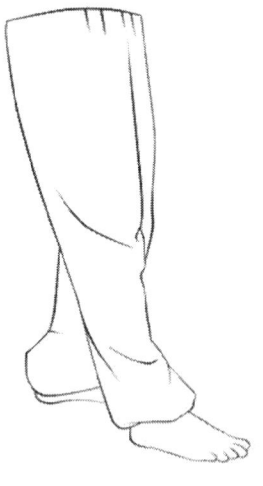

1.

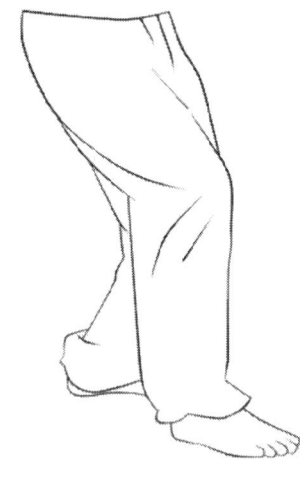

2.

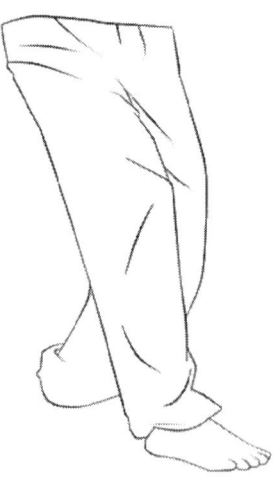

3.

The knees

14. 膝要抱 Hold the knees.

16. 腿要屈 Bend the legs.

Holding the knees means preventing them from collapsing in or out.

This kind of holding is more evident in a fixed position, such as a (narrow) horse stance in which the inside of the knees embrace an imaginary horse, and at the same time are pushed outwards. It is essentially the same thing, except while circle walking the stance is very narrow, and the feet are constantly shifting positions.

Circle walking demands that the knees bend, how far depends on the skill, and needs of the practitioner.

Many people try and bend their knees too much. If you want to walk upright then a knee bend sufficient to lower your head about three to six inches (about half it's height) is plenty for most people. The deeper you go the harder it will be to remain relaxed and the easier it will be to over strain your knees.

Generally when circle walking you want to avoid bobbing up and down. To stay smooth and level demands that you bend the knee of the weighted foot when the hip passes over it.

The feet

21. 足要弼 The feet should be jabbing.

22. 趾要扣 The toes should hook

The first line describes the movement of the foot as it extends forward, which is to say that there is ankle plantar flexion.

Figure 4. the feet should jab

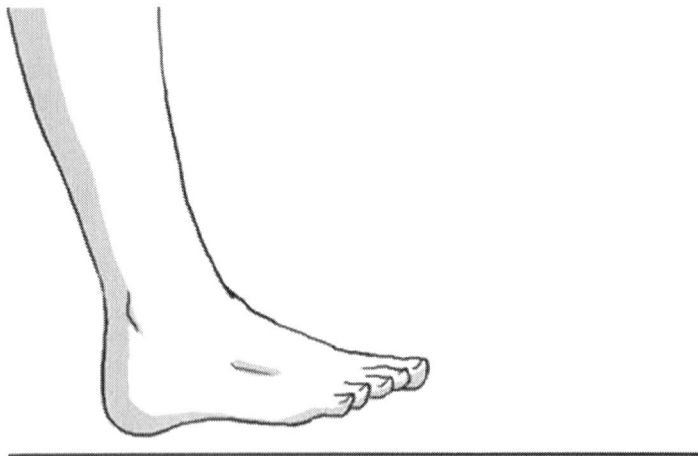

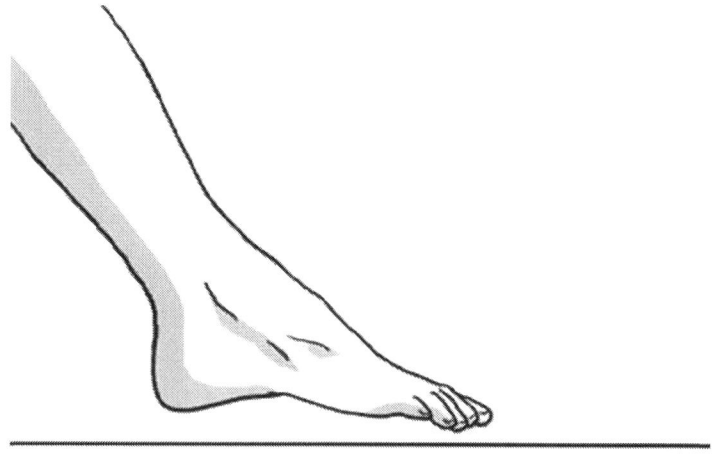

The second line describes the action of the toes as the foot makes contact with the ground — they should hook or grasp the ground slightly.

It is a coincidence but these two lines also describe foot placement. While there are many variations of this in different styles of *Bagua*, in the *Gao* style the inner foot goes straight ahead — it jabs, while the outer foot hooks inwards. The hooked angle of the outside foot is created by turning the toes of the foot inwards rather than turning the heel outwards.

The end result is that as you walk you can imagine two parallel rails on the ground. These rails do not follow a perfect circle, they have distinct if slightly angled corners. the position of each corner is the planted position of the outside foot.

These imaginary rails are usually no wider than a fist width apart (people with large hips and thighs may need to make this wider). As one foot passes the other you can easily check the distance, and the direction of the planted foot will give the direction to follow.

The degree of hooking with the outside foot will vary, less if you walk a circle with a larger diameter, more angle if the diameter is smaller. Once the outside foot has completed its step the line of the inside foot should extend to touch the outside foot.

Generally aim to keep the feet parallel to the ground as they move.

Figure 5. the inside foot moves on a line parallel to the outside foot

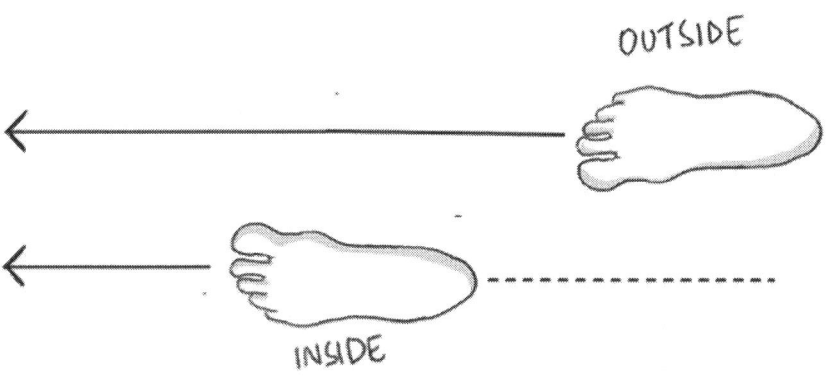

Figure 6. The outside foot hooks inwards

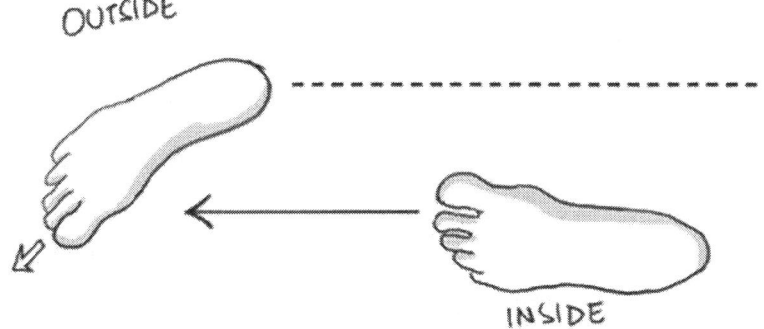

Figure 7. inside and outside feet combined

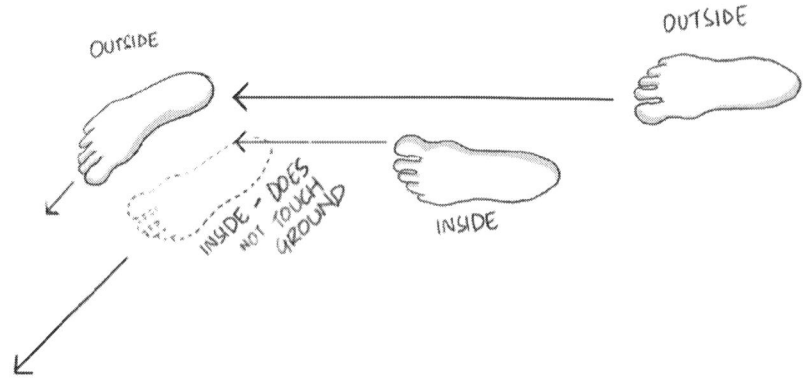

Bagua involves both hooking (*koubu*) and swinging steps (*baibu*) where the toes turn outwards. During *Gao* style circle walking the emphasis is on the hook step, which mimics outflanking an opponent. Swinging steps are found in changes of direction, and are also very integral to the *Hotien* linear forms of *Gao* style *Bagua*.

The arms

15. 臂要伸 Stretch your arms.

17. 腕要塌 The wrists should sink.

18. 指要撑 The fingers should firmly separate.

19. 指對肘 The fingers are aligned with the elbows.

20. 肘掩心 The elbows cover the heart.

Consider these instructions alongside the section on the torso. Overall they describe a way to hold the arms so that they can be connected to body to transfer force back and forth from centre to edges.

This is achieved by an overall stretch in the arms out to the fingertips, the individual lines show ways to increase that stretch.

Imagine a string tied to a nail on each end of the board. You can increase tension on the string by either making the board longer, or the string shorter (contracting your muscles).

Another way would be to hammer some nails into that board in a gentle zigzag then hook the string over alternate sides of each nail. This is equivalent to sinking and twisting individual joints along the arms.

In practice the feeling of stretch is most evident in hands and forearms. The arms should be extended outwards from the body and should feel slightly stretched. This is helped by the other suggestions for the shoulders, elbows, wrists and fingers.

The wrists drop relative to the fingers. The sinking of the wrists requires that the forearms rotate relative to the elbows, which adds to the stretch of the arms and also contributes to their overall firmness.

The fingers are not limp, there is extension and awareness right to their tips. There is space between each finger.

In the way I was taught the fore and middle finger stretch straight up, while the ring finger, little finger and thumb squeeze towards each other slightly, with the space between the thumb and forefinger stretched open. This creates a hollowing of the palm. I realize different schools teach different hand shapes.

Figure 8. Palm shape

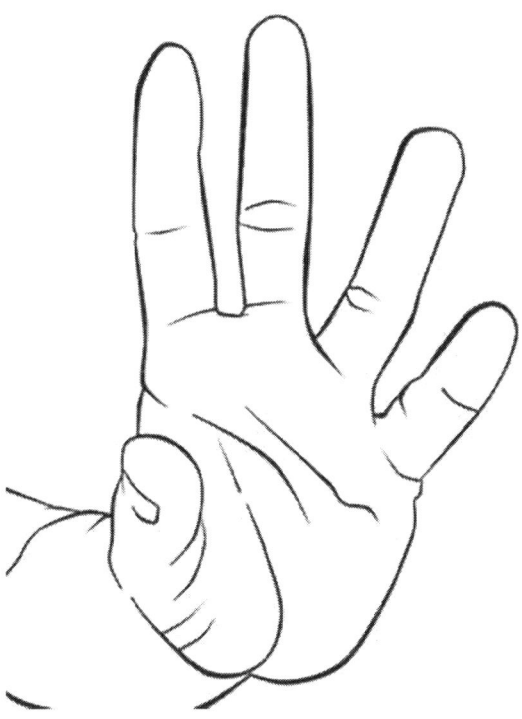

However irrespective of hand shape, one key concept remains universal. The fingers are the ends of the arms so the degree of engagement of the fingers has a significant effect on the overall stretch and connection through the arms. I consider the fingers like the tuning knobs on a guitar, they go a long way to tuning the correct tension.

The elbows sink, the fingers lift, another complementary relation. Also just as the elbows sink to allow the shoulders to transfer force along the arms, the elbows push towards the fingers.

The fingers pointing to the elbow also means that the rear middle finger points towards the front elbow. The rear elbow is low and stays close to the body (covers the heart). This means the elbows have to drop, which helps the shoulders to relax. This also serves as a contrast to the *Santishi* posture of *Xingyiquan* in which the rear elbow does rotate out to some extent.

There is a distortion among many *Bagua* and *Xingyi* practitioners who hold their elbows some distance from their bodies. This is usually a result of having had very overweight teachers somewhere in their lineage. In a fat person the belly prevents their elbow from dropping. This is not something to be imitated in practitioners of healthy weight.

Stepping Methods

23. 步要趨 The steps should be extended

24. 行要穩 The walking should be stable.

The extension of the step refers to the final phase of movement of the forward foot. The idea is that there is some extra effort to push the foot a little further by letting the rear knee drop to push the front foot a little further. Doing this makes walking harder work, and the idea behind it is to build power in the legs that can be transferred to the upper body.

Figure 9.Extend the step – go as far as you can then push a little further

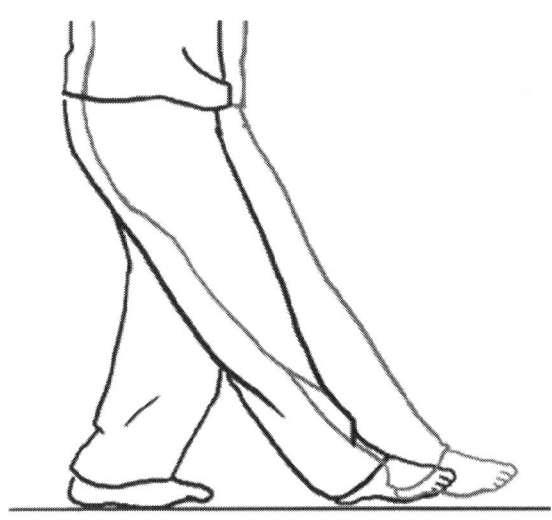

That something as obvious as walking should be stable is stated shows that there are more specific meanings to the phrase.

The first is that the body should be stable on one leg, during each transition of weight, it also refers to not bobbing up and down during each step.

If the body is stable when the ankles are close and the unweighted foot is parallel to the ground at this point then it forces the body to sit — connecting to the lines about holding the *dantien* and lifting the anus.

Stability can also refer to how the foot is lifted and placed. There is a lot to be said for lifting the foot flat so that the whole sole leaves the ground simultaneously. This develops active foot strength, ankle and Achilles tendon flexibility. The foot can be replaced either in a similar manner, or skimming down with the ball of the foot contacting the ground first.

I suggest to start that you practise a firm step, with little or no noise. If balance is difficult to start with slide the ball of your moving foot along the ground until you no longer need the tactile feedback to stay stable.

When it comes to stepping there is considerable variability between styles, and within styles. Each of the many methods for stepping has it's own logic and development goal. Don't get hung about whether a style is right or wrong, focus on what you need to work on. As you progress you can get curious about why others do it differently. Some variations include lifting the foot high as it steps, sliding the foot along the ground, either flat or ploughing with the heel.

Though this is not referred to in these lines it's probably worth mentioning now that walking speed can vary. Sometimes it's great to walk really slowly, though it's important, or vital to also be able to walk quickly. The transfer of weight into the foot needs to have the potential to be quick and clear.

Fast walking while holding all the requirements above is hard work, and good conditioning.

Generally it is easier to walk at a moderate speed.

Very slow walking shows weaknesses in legs and balance.

As the tempo increases the ability to smoothly channel momentum becomes tested, as do any flaws in body rhythm, or the ability to use the body as a coordinated whole.

Use the different walking speeds to expose and work on your weaknesses.

Postures

Most schools of *Baguazhang* have eight fixed postures used to develop the body while circle walking, often referred to as *bamuzhang* (eight mother palms). Some schools have a great many more, but eight is the most common, and the eight tend to be similar though rarely identical.

Different schools sometimes have special forms that they use to change from walking in one direction to walking in the other direction. These forms can be quite interesting however the essential is to hold the postures.

How much emphasis is put on fixed posture walking varies from school to school. In some schools fixed posture walking for a number of *years* is a prerequisite to moving forms.

Our school tends to be moderate. The first two or three postures are used to introduce students to circle walking before moving forms such as single palm change are introduced.

The thinking behind this is that beginners tend not to have the physical awareness or patience to go deeply into fixed posture practice. As experience accumulates it gets easier to appreciate how these postures help understanding with body use and power.

Also we tend to emphasize focus over duration in these postures. The goal is not to hold each one for hours, but rather find the correct position efficiently and through appropriate relaxation feel the work involved after just a few circles on each side.

1. Lower Pressing Posture 下按式　　Xia An Shi

In the first the hands press palm down at about the level of the hips, the fingers point forwards. A common variation is to walk with the palms down and the fingers pointing towards each other.

The intention is to push the palms down. Keep the elbows almost straight and the upper back smooth (do not retract the shoulder blades). The head presses upwards to counter the downward push of the palms.

Figure 10. lower pressing posture

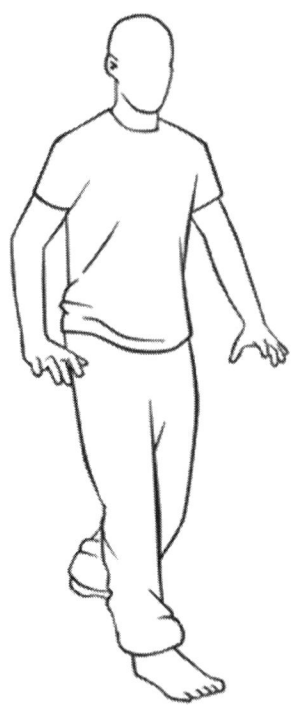

2.   Holding The Taiji Posture 抱太極   Bao Taiji

In the second posture the hands are held at chest height, thumbs slightly lower than the little fingers, the palms curved. Keep the elbows dropped.

The intention is to focus the force of the body in the space between the hands.

Figure 11. Holding the Taiji posture

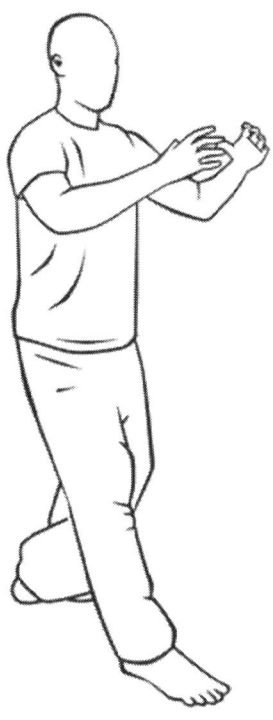

3. *Floating Wood Palm*   漂木掌   *Piao Mu Zhang*

In the third posture the hands are held out to the sides slightly below shoulder level, with the elbows slightly in front of the line of the chest. The arms should feel heavy, the fingers slightly stretched.

The intention is split between the two palms as if there was something balanced in each of them.

Figure 12. Floating wood palm

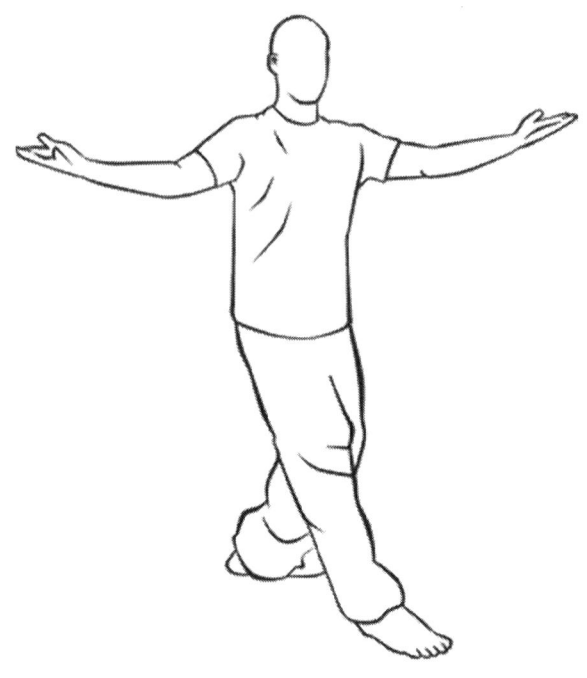

4. *Support Spear Palm* 托槍式 *Tuo Qiang Shi*

The fourth is the first of the twisted postures. Twisted postures are harder to manage as the head does not look in the same direction as you walk.

In the fourth posture the inside hand remains in essentially the same place as the third posture, though slightly higher. The outside hand pushes up above it, about a forearm length diagonally towards the head. The overall effect is of holding a basket ball/beach ball in the palms. The intention focuses the strength of the body into this space.

Pay attention to keeping the outside arm shoulder and elbow as low as possible. Imagine that the outside hand pushing into the centre powers the turning of the body as you walk.

Figure 13. Support spear palm

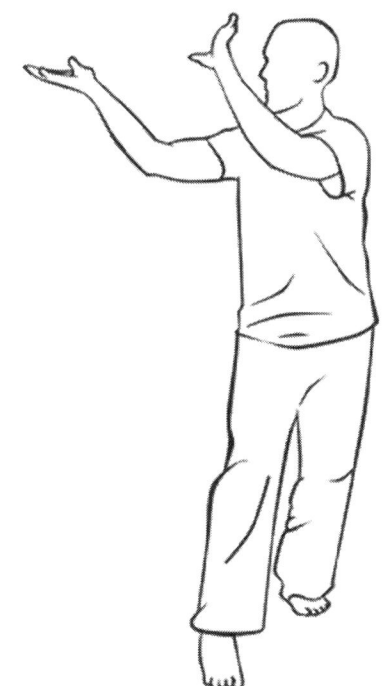

5. *Upper and Lower Vertical Palm* - 上下立掌 *Shang Xia Li Zhang*

(or Piercing Heaven Hitting Earth - 指天打地 Zhi Tian Da Di)

Push the inside arm up so the forearm is vertical and there is a twisting through to the fingertips. Push the outside fingertips diagonally down across the body and into the circle. The combination of stretching up and down engages the spine, which should press backwards. Use the 'urging of the outside hand to power the rotation as you walk.

Figure 14 Upper and lower vertical palm

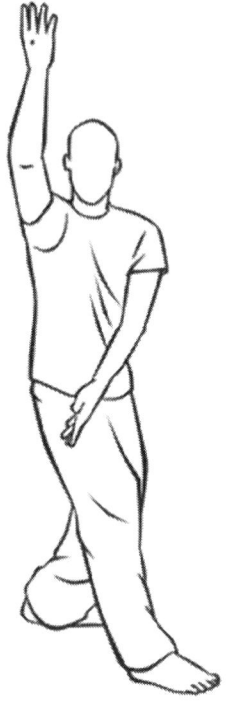

6. *Double Holding Palm* - 雙抱掌 *Shuang Bao Zhang*

(or White Monkey Offers Peaches - 白猴獻桃 Bai Hou Xian Tao)

Pull the elbows together, push the palms into the centre, and pull your fingers down towards the ground. To do this you will need to protract (separate) your shoulder blades, and you can continue this by curving your upper back.

The feeling in this curved posture is that the palms are supported from the kidney/lower back area via the forearms.

This posture encourages a higher lifting of the foot as you walk.

Figure 14 Double holding palm

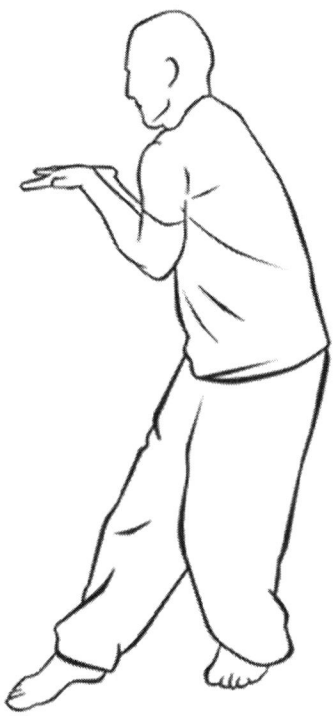

7. Double Crashing Palm - 雙撞掌 Shuang Zhuang Zhang

Pull your elbows apart to create a horizontal line across both forearms with the palms facing down. The head is lifted and the shoulder blades retracted.

Figure 15 Double crashing palm

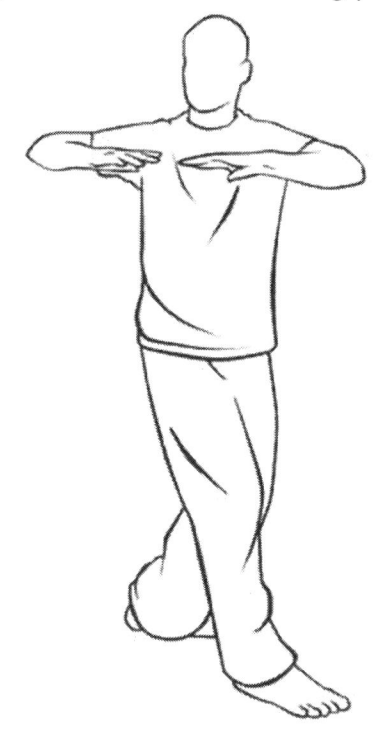

8. *Turning Palm* 轉環掌   *Zhuan Huan Zhang*

The eighth posture is the familiar circle walking shape. Many of the requirements have been described already, so you may want to re-read the sections above.

To recapitulate − the front hand index finger is eye level and vertical and presses into the centre of the circle. The outside hand is about a hand's breadth from the inside elbow. The degree to which you press towards the centre of the circle with the lower hand determines the degree to which the body twists inwards.

Figure 16. Turning palm

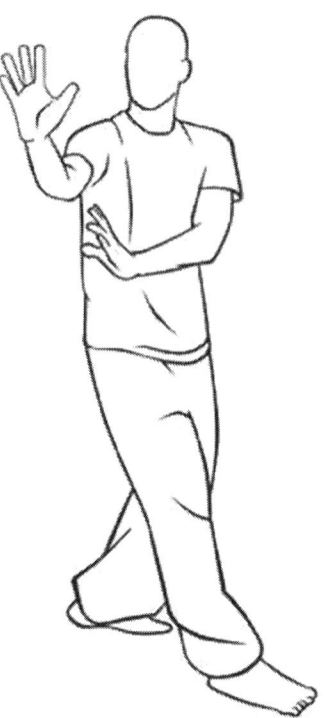

The intention in this posture is less straightforward than the others. The eyes gaze towards the index finger, both hands press towards the centre, while the spine presses away from the centre. The attention outwards from the spine links to the intention inwards of the eyes and palms with an awareness of front-back-side-side.

I'd simply say that the intention creates a sphere around the body, but this is not an excuse to start hallucinating energy balls.

The intention is just on being aware of owning the all the space within the sphere, and in a similar way to the space of the whole circle.

Single Palm Change – Danhuanzhang
單換掌

Single palm change is the key movement of many styles of *Baguazhang*, and the only moving form that I shall introduce in this book.

According to many the founder of *Baguazhang* taught three movements to all of his students as part of the foundation for their training. These movements were single palm change, double palm change and smooth palm change.

When I describe single palm change as a key movement what I mean is that it contains all the movement ingredients of other forms. It has *kou* and *bai* steps, horizontal, diagonal and vertical circles, opening and closing, turning away from the centre and turning back, separating force and crossing force.

Single palm change is worthy of a book in itself — which is why I'm writing one.

As ever different styles have different ways to practise single palm change. Some add in elements like a sharp piercing in *Liang* style, or sitting deeply into various steps.

The version that I present is a very 'average' version. It has no tempo changes, it is not too deep and not too high.

As you move through the steps presented below, take your time. Imagine that you are moving against a resistance, that your hands are pushing against a force opposite to their direction of travel.

Do not limit this to your hands. Ask how your hands are supported by the other parts of your body. How do your elbows support your hands? How do your shoulders support your elbows and hands? How does your spine support your shoulders?

Consider this all the way down to your feet.

To keep the movement balanced it is not just your hands that are engaged this way. If you can support force in the direction of travel with your hands correctly, you can also support force with other parts of the body from other directions.

If you can support force forwards with the front hand, consider also how you can support force in the opposite direction with your back.

If you can support force to the outside with the exterior surface of your arms, can you simultaneously support force to the inside with the interior surface?

And (this is quite a big *and)* can you do all of this while remaining flexible relaxed and not stiff in your body?

Start the sequence with the last of the eight mother palms as in the drawing below.

Figure 17. turning palm

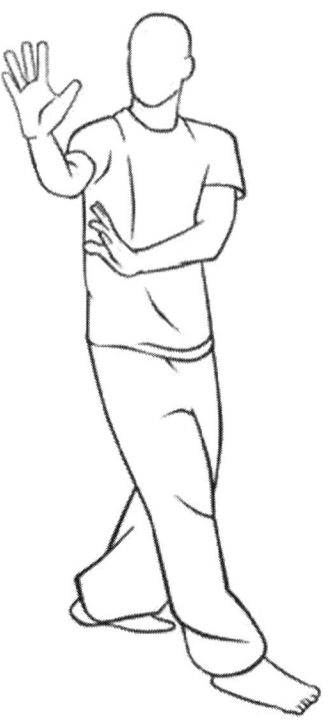

1. Shift the weight forward into the right leg, pick up the left foot, and take a *kou* (toe in or hook) step in front of the right leg. The upper body remains largely unchanged externally. The step and the right hand are coordinated however. It is the pushing into the centre of the left hand that pulls the left foot around.

In this posture there is a greater sense of the hands pushing forwards away from the centre line, and this needs to be balanced by a greater sense of pushing the spine backwards. The result is stretch through the back of the body, running along the outside of the arms and back/outside of the legs.

In this position there is a clear, strong *kou* step, with both feet turned towards each other.

Figure 18.

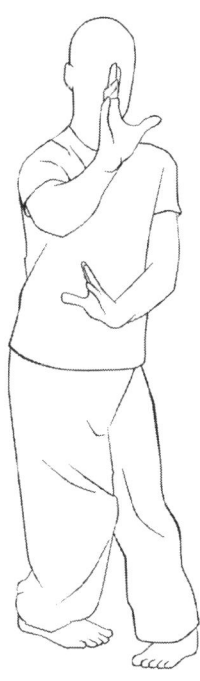

2. Shift the weight into the left foot and lift the right heel, then turn the waist to the right, continuing until you have turned through 180°. The right hand turns so that the fingers are horizontal and the palm faces

out. The left hand pushes down slightly below and to the front of the left hip.

So that you finish in a comfortable position pick up the right foot and place it flat pointing forward with a fist width between the heels, and pointing straight forwards. The right foot also advances slightly. Rotate the left leg inwards as much as is necessary for you to feel stable and comfortable. The left[foot will be turned about about 30° to the right foot.

Figure 19.

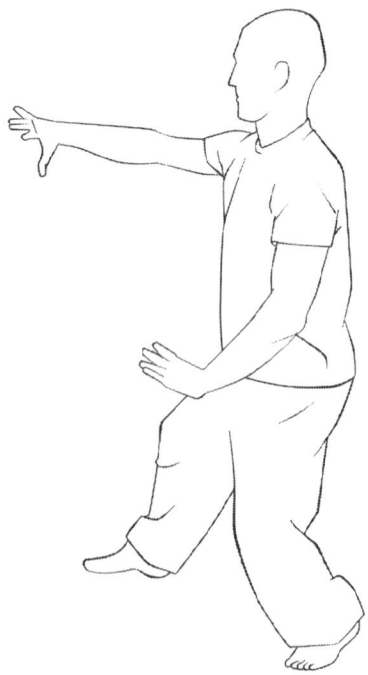

This step is powered partly by a release of the stretch across the back developed in step 1. The pushing down of the left hand supports a sense of pushing forward with the right palm. Keep a sense of settling the weight down and while lifting the spine and expanding the body forwards and back, left and right.

Here the right foot moves in an arc to the outside and so can be considered a *bai*/swing step even though the end position of the foot is straight head.

In terms of circles this step involves a horizontal turn/circle.

3. Shift the weight forward and step past the right foot with the left foot. Keep the left foot pointing straight ahead and the weight in the right leg. Turn the hips to the right and turn the right foot out while maintaining the knee in the same direction as the foot. The right hand remains largely in place while the left palm pushes horizontally under the right armpit.

In this position we have returned to a 'back stretch' similar in some ways to step one, but rounder. The two palms push in opposite directions parallel to the hips, rather than both pushing in the same direction away from the centre line. Imagine that just as the palms can be stable when pushed along the forearm, a push from the opposite direction on the elbow would also be stable.

Figure 20. transitional posture

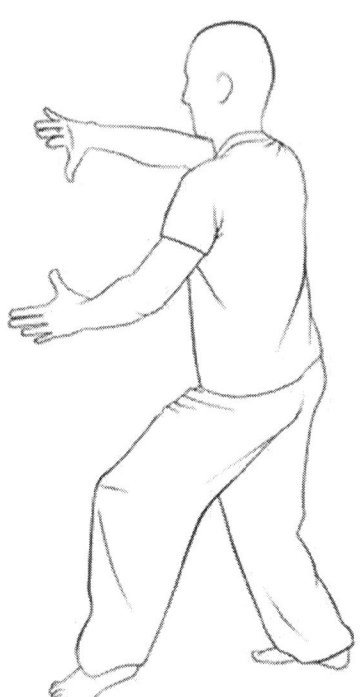

Figure 21. Flower hidden under leaf – front and rear

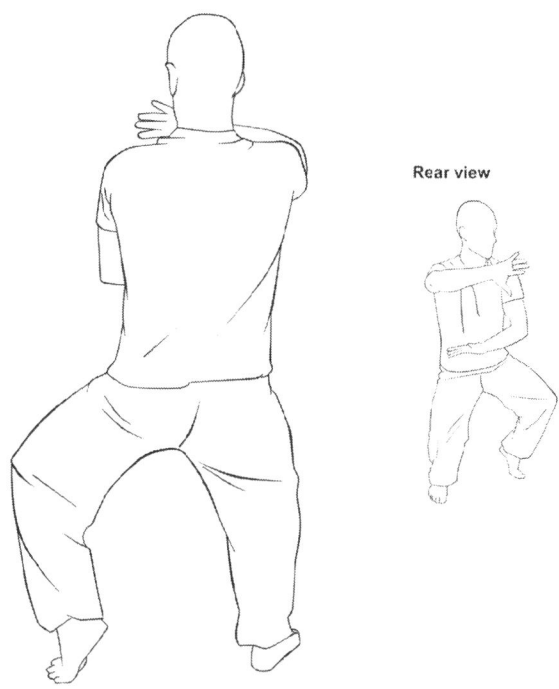

Rear view

Here the right foot turns out clearly into a *bai* step, and the left foot/leg also has a sense of turning out to maintain its straight forwards direction.

Keep the weight in the right foot as it turns outwards. This feels strange to start with and needs some awareness to keep the knee from being twisted especially on a high friction or sticky surface. However this weighted turning is important in developing the body method.

4. Rotate back to the left with the weight still in the right foot. The right fingers drill upwards at a 45° angle and the left hand slides along the underside of the right forearm, continuing the line of movement upwards and outwards.

You can pause with the arms lifted at 45° to vertical, the palms facing in and the right hand on the inside of the left elbow, and the right fingertips around nose level.

In this position one of the key points is the supination (inward turn) of the palms that adds to the stretch and tension throughout the body. You can also stretch the entire body upwards

In terms of circles this step involves a diagonal arc of the hands.

Figure 21.

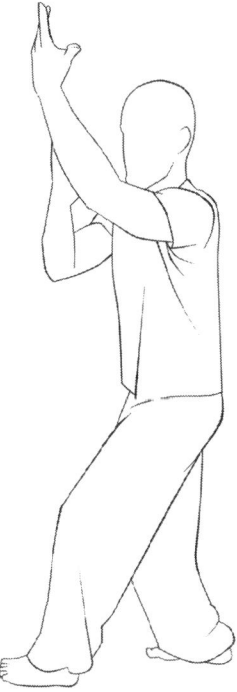

5. Fall back to the original position in 1, allow the hands to turn back, and settle down in the legs and body.

The movement releases the stretch built by the supination of the palms in step 4, and develops the sense of downward power in the body.

In terms of circles this step involves a vertical arc of the hands.

Figure 22. Single palm change in a single image

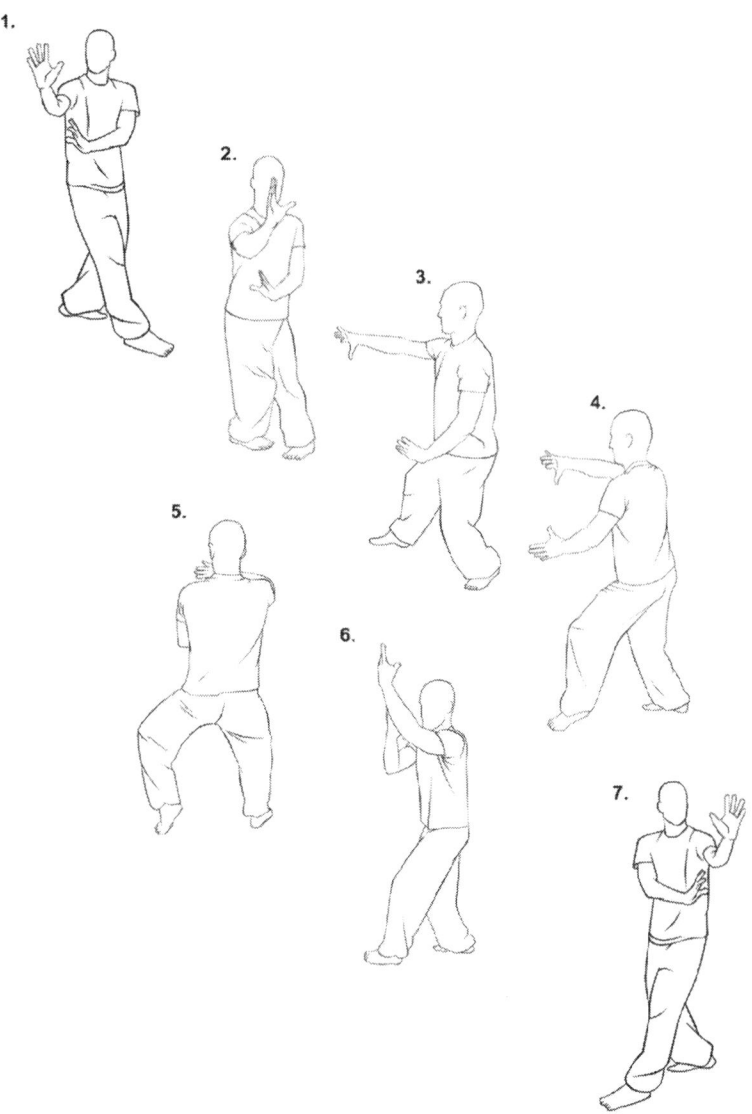

Ways to practise

Circle walking can be practised in many ways, depending on your interest, level, how much time or space you have. There is no single way to practise, no single way to step.

As I mentioned above you cannot practise everything at once. You need to decide what you want to work on, and the choice is wide.

Gao Yisheng gives the advice below.

先練腿 次練身 後練掌

First practice the legs, then train the body, and finally practice the palms.

先求實後求虛，先求重後求輕

First study solid and then study empty. First study heavy, then study light.

尋序漸進，不急功，不燥進.

Proceed in an orderly way and advance step by step, don't be eager for quick success and don't be too eager to advance.

To elucidate the suggestions above.

Arm power depends on the body, body movement depends on the legs. There is to some extent a chicken and egg problem here though. To train the legs correctly, the body needs to be well placed.

Rather than taking this first suggestion as a syllabus to be pursued over months or years, rather take it as advice for a session.

First establish the walking pattern, sit into the legs, place the knees and feet well with each step. Then settle the body into place, and then thirdly add the palms, both in terms of the fixed postures and moving changes.

Studying heavy and solid refers to developing power in the body. My teacher Luo used to quip that the famous *Taiji* saying "use four ounces to deflect a thousand pounds" was only half right. It would be better to say "First have a thousand pounds, *then* use four ounces to deflect a thousand pounds."

Power comes from relaxed, connected heaviness. When the body is nicely connected or unified it can move nimbly and lightly. Heaviness comes from knowing where your body is in space, the relationship between the parts. Lightness comes from sensitivity and the ability to change with the other. First know yourself, then know the other. Once your body is adaptable it can change spontaneously according to the situation.

This idea of changing spontaneously is not some magic formula. Where to go, when to be heavy, when to be light is the result of extended experience in a variety of situations.

In other words partner practise with a variety of different personalities, body types, environments and with different goals in fixed patterns and free sparring.

Finally the advice on proceeding in an orderly manner. Pretty obvious, but important pieces of information are missing. How can you know when you are ready to progress? What are the benchmarks, what is the order?

This is where you really need a trustworthy teacher.

Failing that you have this book, and I'll do my best.

The first thing I want to say is that you will do yourself no favours if you treat circle walking like a workout you need to complete, a question of ticking off the palms and a certain number of circles or steps or changes.

It's not bad to have a program to follow, but skill builds in this area through awareness and attention to correct practice rather than simple repetition.

It does not matter whether you have ten minutes or two hours to dedicate to a practise session, don't rush the process. Quality is king, queen and jack.

So settle your mind and breath as you walk, then work on some specific aspect of circle walking for a while. You can focus on any of the body rules outlined above, until you either feel that it is sufficiently well established for the session, or you can no longer maintain focus.

Remember if you focus on just one body rule while you walk, you can allow the rest of the body to be less precise, the rest of the body does not disappear. Think of it this way, as you tweak the parts, keep an eye on the whole.

If your focus is shot, take a break and start again. If the quality is well established, then move on to another quality or add intensity/complexity to test whether you can maintain what you developed in a more demanding situation.

At the end of a session make some kind of note, mental or otherwise of what you were working on, what was becoming intriguing or frustrating so that you can return to it the next time around.

Oh, and don't torture yourself. Pain and effort can be fun, but if you destroy your enthusiasm for practice so that you feel like you never want to see another circle or step in your life, well you probably are not doing yourself any favours.

A small tip that I have found helps some students — mark your circle, either place something in its centre, use a tree to walk around, or draw a chalk circle on the ground. One aim of circle walking is to develop greater spatial awareness, and this exists to different degrees in different people. Without this I find that many beginners drift, their circles wander.

A big tip is to film yourself. It's usually a shock to see how you look when you walk, but that's the point, what you think you do is not what you actually do. Use the film to get clearer about how you use your body, and the to pick out points to improve. Be your own constructive critic.

Structuring a session

It's possible to practise circle walking in many ways. You can have brief sessions, long sessions, you can walk slowly, you can walk fast, you can practise in a casual way or with intense focus.

My suggestions are

- Set a low minimum time for a session. If you feel like adding more minutes, great.

- Decide the major theme of your session before you start.

- Mentally prepare yourself before you start - relax, feel your body, imagine what you will work on.

- Start gently, incrementally improve your posture and walking method. Adjust your posture as subtly as possible.

- You can start either too relaxed and build up to correct extension, or you can start too tight or extended and back off the tension. The point is do not expect to be instantly 'perfect.

- Do not try and *force* yourself into a posture, feel your self and learn how to get there without force

If you start your circle walking practice with an agitated mind or excessively turbulent emotions it can be helpful to walk fast, the tempo of your steps a reflection of the rhythm of your thoughts. A brisk walk has long been the solution for a difficult state of mind. No need to get too complicated. As your brisk walk works its magic, you will be able to add in the elements of circle walking that you want to practise.

You can divide the body in practice. Sometimes you may choose to focus on the feet or stepping, other days the upper body, other days the arms. This allows you to make clearer distinctions, and also provides a 'way in'. Ideally you want to be aware of and work with the entirety of your body and the space around it, but this is not always possible immediately.

While discipline is important there is a limit to how much you can usefully force your body to do in circle walking. The attitude I recommend is to find a state where in the words of my teacher 'your body teaches you.' It is a balance between your intentions for the session and an openness to new sensations – information from your body that guide your movement, posture and practise.

This is an ongoing process, and what you find in any one session however amazing it may be in the moment is not the end. In fact you may discover at a later date that your prior revelation was very partial, and that some other element is more important.

Power tips, feedback and partners

It is easy to delude yourself in solo practice. Everything feels smooth and cool and if there is insufficient or only very cooperative partner practice it gets easy to think that actual combat will be as easy.

Overly cooperative partner practice can be doubly deluding. Not only do you get to feel like a martial deity, but your partners confirm it. Be warned!!!

With the idea of providing a different kind of feedback to solo walking, I'll just offer a couple of exercises that I like to use when I teach circle walking, especially for people who are just starting.

They both require a partner.

In the first as you circle walk your partner applies a gentle, constant force to your chest. Many beginners tend to lean backwards when stepping forwards, as this is easier on the legs. Others have a slumped posture from desk use.

The forward pressure will prevent you moving forward if your posture is awful, or will require you to use considerable effort to fight against. This level of effort is usually above the threshold of noticing, while the effort required to hold a habitually poor posture is mostly below the threshold — so the added resistance creates a situation where poor habits can be made more evident.

A second exercise that is a bit trickier is for the resisting partner to hold onto the trouser cuffs of the walking partner. It can help with balance and the sense of connection between the feet. It is less easy to gauge the correct level of resistance for the walker. The cuff holder will also have to bend, or squat and duck walk which requires more effort (but can be great for the legs).

Conclusion: Walking in a vacuum

You cannot walk in a vacuum, or at least not for long before you suffocate.

We live in a society which tends value objects, rather than connections. Almost everything can be bought, sold, commoditized.

I see many people treat martial arts in this way, they collect forms, techniques, styles. They expect that a class or two a week will solve their lives.

I catch myself doing that from time to time, scouring the internet for clues, magic bullets, ultimate methods. Circle walking does little good that way. Circle walking is not another possession, or obligation.

Any pleasant activity can become addictive. Something as absorbing and fascinating as circle walking can be addictive, at least in the sense that it provides a space of relative comfort and certainty compared to all the out of control people and events that life presents.

While the capacity to forget everything else during practise is a virtue in circle walking, it works better as a complement to rather than an escape from daily life.

Do not seal off your circle walking from your life, or seal yourself off from your life through circle walking. Just as one aim of circle walking is to unify your body, to connect the feet with our hands, the high with the low, you will do well to use your circle walking to connect to different aspects of your life.

The sensitivity and strength you develop through circle walking will not serve you if you do not use it well. Walk out of doors, walk where you can see the sky, where you can talk to people in the park (even if they can interrupt your practice).

Apply the sensitivity when listening to friends. Use the lightness of movement and balance in other activities whether dance or mixed martial arts, when change comes apply your ability to stand firm or flow with it. Where else can you connect the qualities you develop in circle walking to your life situation?

Circle walking doesn't have beginnings or ends, it does have process.

About the author

I was born in London in 1968, I live in Paris. At the time of writing it is 2015.

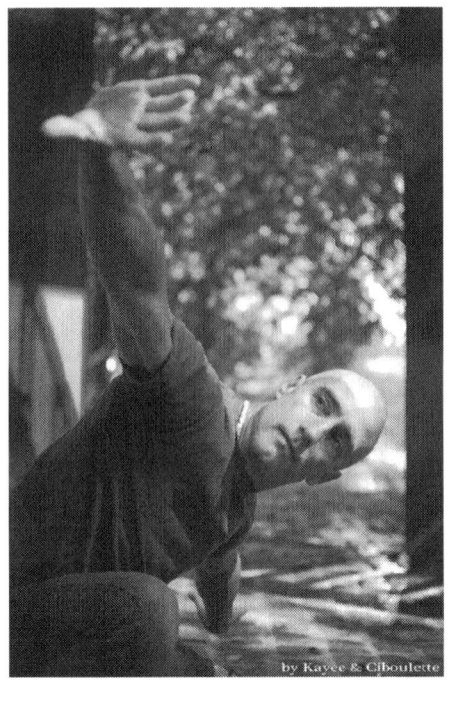

I've been practising *Baguazhang* for twenty four years since I first met my teacher Luo Dexiu in Taiwan in 1991. That is another story. My interest in Chinese martial arts got serious in 1983 when I started to study *Taijiquan* in London. Again that's another story, but it was the one that took me to Taiwan.

For years martial arts were pretty much everything to me. Though I've kept *Bagua* as my martial 'home' I've studied many other arts and traditions over the decades. I used to compete in *sanda*. I've largely lost my taste for being punched in the head and thrown on the ground, I think that can happen with age, but I do know what it's like. I don't write from a flowery or idealistic perspective.

For years martial arts were pretty much everything to me. Now I see them as part of something bigger, part of being human.

It's not so easy to be a healthy human today, urban living, diet, culture all tend to create various distortions. Animal vitality is smothered in domestic settings, childlike curiosity, absorption and play are discouraged in the controlled settings of school and workplace.

This is a big subject. A huge one, it touches on the entirety of our culture and our biology. I am only scratching its surface.

So these days *Baguazhang* is a tool, a practice, a cultural gift that I offer to help to walk the fine line, or broad circle from domestication to wildness and back again.

It's not the only tool I use, but it is a very beautiful one and I am grateful to the people who came before and the ones who will come after.

I'm happy to hear from you! You can write to me at edward@i-bagua.com with your comments, suggestions and requests.

Website

Lots of articles, training tips, ideas and essays that don't fit in books and extracts from past or coming books, not to mention class times and seminar information.

www.I-Bagua.com

Glossary of Chinese

Baguazhang 八卦掌 eight trigram palm

baibu 擺步 swinging step — a step that involves an exterior rotation of the foot

bamuzhang 八母掌 eight mother palms — the fixed hand positions of *baguazhang*

bu 步 a step or stance

dantien 丹田 Literally 'elixir field' in martial arts usually refers to the centre of mass in the lower abdomen, between the lower back, perineum and navel

danhuanzhang 單換掌 Single palm change – the key posture in many styles of Baguazhang

dao 道 Way or process

Gao Yisheng 高義盛 the founder of Gao style Bagua

Hotien 後天 post heaven – refers to an arrangement of the trigrams from the book of changes or Yijing

koubu 扣步 hook step – a step in which the foot rotates inwards

Liang Zhenpu 梁振蒲 the founder of Liang style Bagua

Luo Dexiu 羅德修 the author's teacher

qi 氣 breath and intrinsic quality

sanda 散打 freefighting – also a combat sport that involves punches kicks and throws

santishi 三體勢 three bodies power – a key posture of the martial art Xingyiquan

Taiji 太極 literally 'great pole' the idea that opposites are constantly combined and interchanging. A key idea in Chinese culture.

Taijiquan 太極拳 a martial art named after *Taiji*

xiantien 先天 pre heaven – an arrangement of the trigrams from the classic of change or *Yijing*

Xingyiquan 形意拳 – Form intention boxing, a Chinese martial art often associated with *Baguazhang*

Yijing 易經 the classic of change – a key text of Chinese culture

Links

You already have my website here is my Amazon Author page,
the I-Bagua Facebook page
and here I am on Twitter

Other books by Edward Hines

Beginning Bagua

Moving into Stillness

Coming soon:

Single palm change − a guide to Baguazhang's key movement

The book of Baguazhang basics − big, beautiful and bulshit free

The applied circles of Baguazhang

Printed in Great Britain
by Amazon